THE PHILOSOPHY OF SIBPALKI

A Journey Towards Mastery: From Basic Principles to Advanced Techniques

KAMERON JALEN

Table of Contents

Introduction

SIBPALKI is a traditional Korean martial art that focuses on self-defense techniques and combat skills. SIBPALKI has roots in ancient Korean martial arts, integrating techniques from various styles and emphasizing practical self-defense. It has evolved over centuries, influenced by both Korean culture and other martial arts.

Techniques:

• **Striking**: SIBPALKI includes various striking techniques, such as punches, kicks, and knee strikes.

• **Joint Locks**: The art emphasizes joint locks and throws, allowing practitioners to control an opponent effectively.

• **Self-Defense**: Techniques are designed for real-world self-defense situations, making it practical for everyday application.

Training:

• **Physical Conditioning**: Practitioners engage in physical conditioning to enhance strength, flexibility, and endurance.

• **Forms (Hyung)**: Training often includes practicing forms, which are predefined patterns of movements that help develop technique and focus.

• **Sparring**: Controlled sparring sessions allow practitioners to apply techniques in a dynamic setting.

Philosophy:

• **Discipline and Respect**: Like many martial arts, SIBPALKI emphasizes discipline, respect for instructors and peers, and the importance of mental focus.

- **Self-Improvement**: Practitioners often seek personal growth, confidence, and self-awareness through their training.

Modern Practice:

• **Schools and Associations**: SIBPALKI is taught in various martial arts schools worldwide, with instructors trained in the tradition.

• **Competitions**: Some practitioners participate in competitions, showcasing their skills in forms and sparring.

SIBPALKI offers a comprehensive approach to martial arts, focusing on practical self-defense while promoting physical fitness and mental discipline.

Key Principles And Values

The key principles and values of SIBPALKI reflect its philosophical foundation and approach to martial arts. Here are some of the core principles and values associated with SIBPALKI:

Key Principles:

- **Self-Defense**: The primary focus of SIBPALKI is self-defense. Techniques are designed to help practitioners protect themselves effectively in real-world situations.

- **Practical Application**: Emphasis on techniques that can be used in everyday life. Training scenarios often replicate realistic confrontations.

- **Fluidity and Adaptability**: Practitioners learn to adapt their techniques based on the opponent's movements and actions, fostering a fluid style of combat.

• **Integration of Techniques**: SIBPALKI incorporates various martial arts techniques, emphasizing a comprehensive skill set that includes striking, grappling, and joint locks.

Core Values:

• **Discipline**: Consistent training and dedication are essential. Practitioners develop self-control and perseverance through regular practice.

• **Respect**: Respect for instructors, fellow practitioners, and the art itself is fundamental. This fosters a positive training environment and community.

• **Humility**: Practitioners are encouraged to maintain humility, recognizing that there is always more to learn and improve.

• **Confidence**: Through training, practitioners build self-confidence, which extends beyond martial arts and influences their daily lives.

• **Focus and Mindfulness**: Training encourages mental focus and mindfulness, helping practitioners to concentrate on their techniques and the present moment.

• **Community and Brotherhood**: SIBPALKI fosters a sense of belonging and camaraderie among practitioners, promoting a supportive environment for growth and learning.

• **Physical Fitness**: Emphasizing physical conditioning and health, SIBPALKI encourages practitioners to maintain a healthy lifestyle.

• **Lifelong Learning**: The pursuit of knowledge and skills in martial arts is seen as a lifelong journey, promoting continuous personal development.

These principles and values contribute to the holistic approach of SIBPALKI, making it not just a martial art but a way of life that promotes personal growth, self-awareness, and a sense of responsibility toward oneself and others.

CHAPTER 1: THE FUNDAMENTALS OF SIBPALKI

Stances And Postures

In SIBPALKI, stances and postures are fundamental to executing techniques effectively and maintaining balance, power, and readiness. Here are some of the key stances and postures commonly practiced:

<u>Key Stances:</u>

• **Chamber Stance (Gyeong-nyeon Seogi)**: A preparatory stance where the hands are positioned near the body, ready to react. This stance promotes awareness and readiness for movement.

• **Front Stance (Ap Seogi)**: A stable and strong stance with one foot forward, knees bent, and weight distributed evenly. It is used for both offensive and defensive techniques, providing a solid base for strikes.

• **Back Stance (Dwi Seogi)**: The weight is primarily on the back leg, with the front leg extended forward. This stance allows for quick retreats and counterattacks, offering stability while maintaining distance from the opponent.

• **Horse Riding Stance (Juchum Seogi)**: A low and wide stance with feet parallel and knees bent. This stance is commonly used in training for strength and endurance, and it is often utilized when executing certain strikes or blocks.

• **Cat Stance (Beom Seogi)**: A transitional stance where the weight is primarily on the back leg, with the front foot lightly touching the ground. This stance allows for quick movements and changes in direction.

• **Cross Stance (Kyocha Seogi)**: A stance where one foot crosses in front of the other, often used in transitions and specific techniques. It offers mobility and the ability to shift weight quickly.

<u>Postures:</u>

• **Guard Position**: A defensive posture where the hands are raised to protect the head and body. This position prepares the practitioner to block incoming attacks and respond with strikes.

• **Low Guard**: Hands are positioned lower than the guard position, allowing for low strikes and quick transitions to other techniques.

• **Ready Position**: A neutral stance with feet shoulder-width apart and hands relaxed, signaling readiness for action without aggression.

Importance of Stances and Postures:

• **Balance and Stability**: Proper stances provide a strong foundation, allowing for effective movement, striking, and defensive actions.

• **Power Generation**: Many techniques in SIBPALKI rely on the body's mechanics, and stances help in generating power through proper alignment and movement.

• **Speed and Agility**: Correct postures facilitate quick transitions and movements, enabling practitioners to respond effectively in dynamic situations.

• **Mental Focus**: Maintaining specific stances encourages practitioners to be mindful of their body position and overall awareness in training and combat scenarios.

Training in stances and postures involves repetition and refinement, often integrated into forms (hyung) and sparring drills. Mastery of these fundamentals is crucial for effective technique execution and overall performance in SIBPALKI.

Basic Footwork

Basic footwork in SIBPALKI is essential for maintaining balance, mobility, and effectiveness during techniques. Good footwork allows practitioners to close distances, evade attacks, and create openings for strikes. Here are some key aspects of basic footwork:

<u>Key Footwork Techniques:</u>

• **Step Forward (Ap Seung)**: A simple forward movement to close the distance with an opponent. The lead foot steps forward, followed by the back foot to maintain balance and readiness.

• **Step Backward (Dwi Seung)**: A backward movement used to create distance or evade an attack. The practitioner steps back with the rear foot, then brings the lead foot back to maintain a stable stance.

- **Lateral Step (Yeo Seung)**: Side-stepping to the left or right helps in evading attacks or repositioning oneself. The practitioner moves one foot sideways, followed by the other, maintaining a stable base.

- **Cross Step (Kyocha Seung)**: A technique used to quickly change angles or position. One foot crosses in front of the other, allowing for quick transitions between stances or to evade an opponent's attack.

- **Slide Step (Myeong Seung)**: A quick and smooth movement where one foot slides into a new position without losing balance. This technique helps maintain distance while preparing to strike or defend.

- **Pivot (Jjeon Seung)**: A rotational movement that allows the practitioner to change direction while maintaining a stance.

The lead foot pivots, enabling the body to turn and face a different angle.

Importance of Footwork

• **Balance and Stability**: Good footwork keeps practitioners grounded and stable during movement, reducing the risk of falling or being off-balance when executing techniques.

• **Mobility and Agility**: Practicing footwork enhances speed and the ability to move quickly in any direction, which is crucial in both offensive and defensive situations.

• **Distance Management**: Effective footwork allows practitioners to control the distance between themselves and their opponent, enabling them to engage or disengage as needed.

• **Timing and Rhythm**: Footwork helps develop a sense of timing and rhythm in combat, allowing practitioners to anticipate and react to their opponent's movements.

Practice Drills:

To improve footwork, practitioners often engage in specific drills, including:

• **Footwork Patterns**: Repeatedly practicing basic movements in various combinations to build muscle memory and fluency in transitions.

• **Shadow Fighting**: Practicing footwork and techniques without an opponent, focusing on movement, balance, and form.

• **Partner Drills**: Working with a partner to practice moving in response to their actions, helping to develop reactive footwork.

• **Obstacle Courses**: Setting up cones or markers to navigate through, enhancing agility and spatial awareness while moving.

By focusing on these basic footwork techniques, practitioners of SIBPALKI can enhance their overall effectiveness and confidence in both training and self-defense scenarios.

Breathing Techniques

Breathing techniques play a crucial role in SIBPALKI, as they enhance performance, focus, and overall well-being. Proper breathing can help practitioners maintain energy levels, manage stress, and improve concentration. Here are some key breathing techniques commonly practiced in SIBPALKI:

<u>Key Breathing Techniques</u>

• **Diaphragmatic Breathing**: Also known as abdominal or belly breathing, this technique involves inhaling deeply through the nose, allowing the diaphragm to expand, and filling the lungs fully.

How to Practice:

1. Stand or sit comfortably, place one hand on your chest and the other on your abdomen.
2. Inhale deeply through the nose, focusing on expanding the abdomen rather than the chest.
3. Exhale slowly through the mouth, allowing the abdomen to fall.
4. **Benefits**: Increases oxygen intake, promotes relaxation, and helps to reduce stress.

- **Rhythmic Breathing**: This technique involves coordinating breath with movements, such as inhaling during specific actions (like executing a strike) and exhaling during others (like a block or retreat).

How to Practice: During training, practice inhaling when preparing for a technique and exhaling as you execute it.

Benefits: Enhances timing, focus, and efficiency in movements, while also providing a calming rhythm.

- **Four-Count Breathing**: This technique involves inhaling for a count of four, holding the breath for four counts, exhaling for four counts, and then holding the exhale for another four counts.

How to Practice:

1. Inhale through the nose for a count of four, hold for four, exhale through the mouth for four, and hold for four.

2. **Benefits**: Helps regulate breathing, increases lung capacity, and calms the mind.

• **Forceful Exhalation (Kihap)**: Often used in martial arts, kihap involves a sharp exhalation, typically accompanied by a shout or vocalization during strikes or intense movements.

How to Practice:

1. During training, practice exhaling sharply while executing techniques. This can also be integrated into kihap to enhance power and focus.

2. **Benefits**: Increases energy and power in techniques, helps release

tension, and can intimidate an opponent.

• **Visualization with Breath**: Combining breath with visualization can enhance mental focus and relaxation.

How to Practice:

1. While breathing deeply, visualize energy flowing through your body, or imagine releasing stress with each exhale.
2. **Benefits**: Improves concentration, promotes mental clarity, and enhances relaxation.

Importance of Breathing Techniques:

• **Oxygenation**: Proper breathing techniques increase oxygen intake, essential for physical performance and endurance during training and combat.

• **Stress Management**: Controlled breathing helps reduce anxiety and stress, allowing practitioners to maintain calmness and focus during challenging situations.

• **Mind-Body Connection**: Breathing techniques enhance awareness of the body and its movements, fostering a deeper connection between mind and body.

• **Energy Control**: Regulating breath helps manage energy levels, ensuring practitioners can maintain stamina throughout training and sparring.

To incorporate breathing techniques into SIBPALKI training:

• **Warm-Up**: Begin sessions with diaphragmatic breathing to promote relaxation and focus.

• **During Techniques**: Consciously apply rhythmic breathing while practicing stances, strikes, and footwork.

• **Cool Down**: End sessions with calming breathing exercises to promote recovery and relaxation.

By integrating these breathing techniques into their practice, SIBPALKI practitioners can enhance their performance, focus, and overall well-being.

CHAPTER 2: BASIC TECHNIQUES

Hand Techniques

Hand techniques in SIBPALKI are essential for effective striking, blocking, and self-defense. These techniques utilize various parts of the hand, including fists, palms, and fingers, to deliver powerful attacks and execute defensive maneuvers. Here's an overview of some fundamental hand techniques used in SIBPALKI:

<u>Key Hand Techniques:</u>

• **Straight Punch (Jireugi)**: A fundamental technique where the fist moves directly toward the target.

Execution:

1. Start from a guard position, extend the arm forward while rotating the fist so that the palm faces down at impact.

2. Engage the core and hips for power, and exhale during the punch.

• **Hook Punch (Hook Jireugi)**: A circular punch aimed at the opponent's head or body, often used in close combat.

Execution:

1. Rotate the shoulder while bringing the fist around in a hooking motion, keeping the elbow bent.
2. Aim for the side of the target and ensure the fist is horizontal upon impact.

• **Uppercut (Eolgul Jireugi)**: An upward punch directed at the opponent's chin or jaw.

Execution:

1. From a guard position, drop the fist slightly before driving it upward towards the target, using the legs and core for power.
2. Keep the elbow close to the body and ensure the wrist is straight upon impact.

• **Palm Strike (Son Chigi)**: A strike using the palm of the hand, effective for close-range self-defense.

Execution:

1. Strike forward with an open palm, aiming for the opponent's nose, chin, or throat, utilizing body weight for power.

• **Back Fist Strike (Deung Jjireugi)**: A quick strike using the back of the fist, typically aimed at the head or face.

Execution:

2. Rotate the shoulder while snapping the arm out, striking with the back of the fist.
3. Maintain a firm wrist and keep the elbow slightly bent.

• **Knife Hand Strike (Sonnal Chigi)**: A strike using the edge of the hand, effective for cutting or targeting vulnerable areas.

Execution:

1. Extend the hand with fingers together and strike downward or sideways, aiming for the neck, collarbone, or side of the head.

- **Hammer Fist (Bong Jjireugi)**: A downward strike using the bottom of the fist, effective against an opponent's head or collarbone.

Execution:

  - Raise the fist and bring it down in a hammering motion, keeping the wrist straight and engaging the core for power.

- **Fingertip Strike (Sonnal Jjireugi)**: A precise strike using the fingertips, often targeting pressure points or vulnerable areas.

Execution:

  - Extend the fingers and strike with the tips towards sensitive areas like the eyes or throat.

<u>**Blocking Techniques:**</u>

• **High Block (Olgul Makki)**: A defensive maneuver used to deflect attacks aimed at the head.

Execution:

- Raise the arm above the head, using the forearm to block while keeping the other hand in a guard position.

• **Middle Block (Maka Makki)**: A technique to block mid-level attacks aimed at the torso.

Execution:

- Bring the forearm horizontally across the body to intercept the incoming attack.

• **Low Block (Arae Makki)**: A defensive technique to protect against low strikes or kicks.

Execution:

- Lower the arm to a horizontal position at hip level, using the forearm to deflect the attack.

<u>Importance of Hand Techniques:</u>

• **Power Generation**: Proper technique allows practitioners to generate maximum power through body mechanics, leading to effective strikes.

• **Versatility**: A variety of hand techniques provide practitioners with multiple options for both offensive and defensive situations.

• **Self-Defense**: Effective hand techniques are essential for personal safety, enabling practitioners to respond quickly to threats.

To master hand techniques in SIBPALKI, practitioners should:

• **Repetition**: Consistently practice each technique to develop muscle memory and precision.

• **Partner Drills**: Work with a partner to practice strikes and blocks, enhancing timing and reaction skills.

• **Shadow Fighting**: Perform techniques in a solo practice to refine form and technique.

By focusing on these hand techniques, SIBPALKI practitioners can enhance their striking skills and overall effectiveness in both training and self-defense scenarios.

Kicking techniques in SIBPALKI are crucial for delivering powerful strikes, maintaining distance, and executing effective self-defense maneuvers. Kicks can target various parts of the opponent's body, including the head, torso, and legs. Here's an overview of the key kicking techniques commonly practiced in SIBPALKI:

Key Kicking Techniques:

- **Front Kick (Ap Chagi)**: A straightforward kick aimed at the opponent's torso or head.

Execution:

2. Lift the knee up, extend the leg forward, and strike with the ball of the foot or the instep.

3. Focus on a quick retraction after the kick to maintain balance and readiness.

• **Roundhouse Kick (Dollyo Chagi)**: A powerful kick delivered in a circular motion, targeting the opponent's head or body.

Execution:

1. Pivot on the supporting foot while lifting the knee and swinging the leg in a circular motion.
2. Strike with the shin or the top of the foot, ensuring proper hip rotation for power.

• **Side Kick (Yeop Chagi)**: A lateral kick aimed at the opponent's body or head, known for its power and effectiveness.

Execution:

1. Turn the supporting foot outward, lift the knee to the side, and extend the leg straight out while striking with the heel or the edge of the foot.

2. Engage the hips for added force, and be ready to retract the leg for balance.

• **Back Kick (Dwi Chagi)**: A powerful kick delivered backward, targeting an opponent directly behind.

Execution:

1. Turn the body slightly, lift the knee, and extend the leg straight back, striking with the heel.

2. This kick is effective for countering attacks from behind.

- **Axe Kick (Geodeureo Chagi)**: A downward striking kick that targets the opponent's head or shoulder.

Execution:

1. Lift the leg high, then bring it down in an axe-like motion, striking with the heel or the ball of the foot.
2. Ensure proper control and balance when executing this kick.

- **Hook Kick (Gul Chagi)**: A kick that uses a hooking motion to strike at the opponent's head or upper body.

Execution:

1. Lift the knee and extend the leg in a hooking motion, striking with the heel or the side of the foot.
2. This kick can be effective for catching an opponent off-guard.

- **Knee Strike (Mureup Chigi)**: While technically not a kick, a knee strike is a powerful technique used in close combat.

Execution:

1. Lift the knee sharply towards the opponent's torso or head, using the knee cap for impact.
2. This technique can be combined with other strikes in close range.

Importance of Kicking Techniques:

- **Power and Reach**: Kicks can generate significant power and allow practitioners to strike from a distance, keeping opponents at bay.

- **Versatility**: Various kicking techniques provide multiple options for both offensive and defensive maneuvers.

• **Balance and Coordination**: Practicing kicks enhances overall balance, coordination, and body control, essential for effective movement in martial arts.

To master kicking techniques in SIBPALKI, practitioners should focus on the following:

• **Repetition**: Regular practice of each kick to develop muscle memory and precision.

• **Target Practice**: Use pads or bags to practice kicks for power and accuracy.

• **Partner Drills**: Work with a partner to practice kicks in a dynamic setting, helping to develop timing and distance management.

• **Shadow Fighting**: Practice kicks in a solo routine to refine form and technique without the distraction of an opponent.

By focusing on these kicking techniques, SIBPALKI practitioners can enhance their striking abilities and overall effectiveness in both training and self-defense scenarios.

Throws And Takedowns

Throws and takedowns are essential components of SIBPALKI, emphasizing balance, technique, and the ability to control an opponent. These techniques can be used to disrupt an opponent's balance, take them to the ground, or gain a dominant position. Here's an overview of the key throws and takedowns commonly practiced in SIBPALKI:

Key Throws and Takedowns

• **Hip Throw (O-goshi)**: A foundational throw where the practitioner uses their hip as a pivot point to throw the opponent.

Execution:

1. Approach the opponent, positioning your body close while gripping their torso.

2. Pivot on the lead foot, turn your hips into the opponent, and use the momentum to lift and throw them over your hip.

• **Shoulder Throw (Seoi Nage)**: A throw that utilizes the shoulder to lift and throw the opponent.

Execution:

1. Step in close to the opponent, turn your body, and place one arm under their armpit while the other arm secures their wrist or shoulder.

2. Pull down while lifting with the shoulder, using your body weight to throw them over your shoulder.

• **Leg Sweep (Ashi Barai)**: A technique that involves sweeping the opponent's legs out from under them.

Execution:

1. Approach the opponent while maintaining balance.
2. Use your foot to sweep one of their legs while pushing them in the opposite direction to unbalance them.

• **Single-Leg Takedown**: A takedown that targets one of the opponent's legs to bring them to the ground.

Execution:

1. Lower your stance and step in toward the opponent's leg, grabbing behind the knee or ankle.

2. Drive forward while lifting the leg and using your body weight to take them down.

• **Double-Leg Takedown**: A takedown that targets both of the opponent's legs, providing a more stable approach.

Execution:

1. Lower your stance and step in toward the opponent, placing your head against their abdomen.
2. Grab behind both knees and lift while driving forward to take them down.

• **Back Takedown (Rear Naked Choke Takedown)**: A technique used to take an opponent down from a rear position.

Execution:

1. Approach from behind and secure an arm around their neck (if applying a choke) or around their waist.
2. Use your weight and leverage to pull them backward or to the side while maintaining control.

• **Suplex**: A throw that involves lifting the opponent off the ground and then throwing them backward.

Execution:

1. Get underneath the opponent's center of gravity while gripping their waist or body.
2. Lift them up and arch your back while throwing them backward.

Importance of Throws and Takedowns:

• **Control**: Throws and takedowns provide the ability to control an opponent's movement and position effectively.

• **Balance Disruption**: These techniques focus on breaking the opponent's balance, making it easier to dominate the fight.

• **Self-Defense**: Understanding how to throw or take down an opponent can be crucial in self-defense situations, allowing practitioners to neutralize threats.

To master throws and takedowns in SIBPALKI, practitioners should focus on the following:

• **Partner Drills**: Practice with a partner to refine technique and ensure safety while learning.

- **Repetition**: Repeatedly practice each throw and takedown to build muscle memory and confidence.

- **Conditioning**: Engage in physical conditioning to build strength, flexibility, and balance, essential for executing these techniques effectively.

- **Controlled Sparring**: Integrate throws and takedowns into controlled sparring sessions to apply techniques in a dynamic environment.

By focusing on these throws and takedowns, SIBPALKI practitioners can enhance their grappling skills and overall effectiveness in both training and self-defense scenarios.

Joint locks and holds are crucial techniques in SIBPALKI, providing practitioners with methods to control, immobilize, or submit an opponent. These techniques leverage the body's natural mechanics and the vulnerabilities of joints to gain a tactical advantage. Here's an overview of key joint locks and holds commonly practiced in SIBPALKI:

<u>Key Joint Locks and Holds:</u>

• **Wrist Lock (Sok Pal Jime)**: A technique that involves twisting or applying pressure to the opponent's wrist joint.

Execution:

1. Secure the opponent's wrist with one hand and use the other hand to push down or twist the wrist.

2. This can cause pain or discomfort, encouraging the opponent to submit or comply.

• **Armbar (Pal Gyeok Jime)**: A joint lock that targets the elbow joint, hyperextending it.

Execution:

1. Position yourself alongside or underneath the opponent's arm.
2. Secure their arm and place your legs around it, then pull their arm down while pushing their elbow up, applying pressure to the joint.

• **Shoulder Lock (Eolgul Jime)**: A technique that targets the shoulder joint, often used to control or submit an opponent.

Execution:

1. Grip the opponent's arm and pull it toward you while applying downward pressure to the shoulder.
2. You can also use your body weight to create leverage and further control their movement.

• **Knee Lock (Mureup Jime)**: A joint lock applied to the knee, often used in grappling situations.

Execution:

1. Position yourself next to the opponent's knee and secure their leg.
2. Apply pressure to the knee joint by twisting or pushing while maintaining control over their body.

- **Finger Lock (Son Jime)**: A lock that targets the fingers, causing pain and forcing compliance.

Execution:

1. Grip one of the opponent's fingers and twist or pull while applying pressure.
2. This technique is useful for control without significant force.

- **Body Lock (Gyeol Jime)**: A hold that involves securing the opponent's body, often used in grappling.

Execution:

1. Wrap your arms around the opponent's torso, using your weight to control their movement.
2. This hold can be combined with other techniques for further control.

• **Rear Naked Choke (Hansoku Jime)**: A submission hold applied from behind that constricts the opponent's airway or blood flow.

Execution:

1. Position yourself behind the opponent, wrap one arm around their neck, and secure the grip with the other arm.
2. Squeeze and apply pressure to create a choke, leading to submission.

<u>Importance of Joint Locks and Holds:</u>

• **Control**: Joint locks and holds allow practitioners to control an opponent's movements effectively, reducing the risk of retaliation.

• **Submissions**: These techniques provide options for forcing an opponent to submit, creating an opportunity to end a confrontation decisively.

• **Self-Defense**: Understanding how to apply joint locks can enhance personal safety, allowing practitioners to neutralize threats without excessive force.

To master joint locks and holds in SIBPALKI, practitioners should focus on the following:

• **Partner Drills**: Work with a partner to practice each joint lock and hold, ensuring safety and proper technique.

• **Repetition**: Regularly practice to develop muscle memory and confidence in executing these techniques.

• **Controlled Sparring**: Integrate joint locks and holds into sparring sessions to apply techniques dynamically and refine timing.

• **Safety Precautions**: Always practice with care, ensuring that partners communicate clearly and respect each other's limits to avoid injury.

By focusing on these joint locks and holds, SIBPALKI practitioners can enhance their grappling skills and overall effectiveness in both training and self-defense scenarios.

CHAPTER 3: SPARRING AND APPLICATION

The Rules Of Sparring

Sparring is an essential aspect of SIBPALKI training, allowing practitioners to apply techniques in a controlled, dynamic environment. To ensure safety, respect, and effective learning, it's important to follow specific rules during sparring sessions. Here's an overview of the key rules of sparring in SIBPALKI:

Key Rules of Sparring

Safety Gear:

• Practitioners must wear appropriate protective gear, including headgear, mouthguards, gloves, shin guards, and chest protectors.

• Ensure that all gear is in good condition and fits properly.

Respect and Sportsmanship:

• Always show respect for your sparring partner, instructors, and the training environment.

• Display good sportsmanship, regardless of the outcome of the sparring match.

Controlled Techniques:

• Sparring should emphasize control rather than aggression. Practitioners must use techniques with precision and awareness of their partner's safety.

• Avoid excessive force, especially in sensitive areas such as the head and neck.

Communication:

• Partners should communicate before, during, and after sparring. Discuss any concerns or limitations to ensure a comfortable experience for both.

• Check in with your partner after rounds to provide feedback and assess their well-being.

Target Areas:

• Clearly define target areas before sparring, such as the head, torso, and legs.

• Strikes to certain areas may be restricted, depending on the sparring level and context (e.g., beginner vs. advanced).

Duration of Rounds:

• Sparring sessions are typically conducted in timed rounds (e.g., 2-3 minutes) with breaks in between.

• This allows practitioners to rest, regroup, and receive feedback from instructors.

No Intent to Injure:

• The primary goal of sparring is skill development, not to harm the opponent. Intentional strikes aimed at causing injury are strictly prohibited.

• Practitioners should stop immediately if a partner appears injured or in distress.

Takedowns and Grappling:

• If allowed, practitioners should apply takedowns and grappling techniques with care, ensuring that their partner's safety is a priority.

• Avoid slamming or dropping your partner unless specified in advanced sparring.

Follow Instructor Guidance:

• Always adhere to the instructions and rules set by the instructor or coach. They may adjust rules based on the skill level and experience of the practitioners.

Respect the Dojo Etiquette:

• Follow the dojo's etiquette regarding entering and leaving the mat, bowing, and addressing instructors and fellow practitioners.

• Maintain a positive and respectful atmosphere throughout the training session.

<u>**Importance of Following Sparring Rules:**</u>

• **Safety**: Adhering to these rules helps minimize the risk of injury and creates a safe training environment for all practitioners.

• **Skill Development**: Sparring rules facilitate a focus on technique, timing, and strategy, allowing practitioners to enhance their skills effectively.

• **Respectful Environment**: Following etiquette and showing respect foster a positive training atmosphere, encouraging growth and camaraderie among practitioners.

By understanding and adhering to the rules of sparring in SIBPALKI, practitioners can ensure a safe and productive training experience. These rules not only protect individuals during sparring but also promote a culture of respect, growth, and shared learning within the martial arts community.

Sparring Techniques

Sparring techniques in SIBPALKI are essential for developing practical skills, timing, and strategy in a dynamic environment. These techniques encompass various offensive and defensive maneuvers, allowing practitioners to apply what they've learned in a controlled sparring setting. Here's an overview of key sparring techniques in SIBPALKI:

<u>Key Sparring Techniques</u>

1. Footwork:

• **Importance**: Good footwork is crucial for maintaining balance, creating distance, and setting up attacks.

Techniques:

• **Lateral Movement**: Step side to side to evade strikes and position yourself for counterattacks.

• **Forward and Backward Movement**: Use quick steps to close the distance or retreat to avoid incoming attacks.

• **Pivoting**: Rotate on the lead foot to change angles and evade strikes while maintaining a solid stance.

2. Striking Techniques:

• **Punches**: Use various punches (straight, hook, uppercut) to target different areas of the opponent's body.

• **Kicks**: Incorporate kicks (front, roundhouse, side) to deliver powerful strikes and maintain distance.

• **Combos**: Combine punches and kicks in sequences to create effective attack patterns and keep your opponent guessing.

3. Defensive Techniques:

• **Blocking**: Use your arms and legs to block incoming strikes effectively.

• **High Block**: Deflect strikes aimed at the head.

• **Middle Block**: Protect against body shots.

• **Low Block**: Guard against low kicks.

• **Parrying**: Redirect incoming strikes away from your body using a quick movement of the hands.

• **Evading**: Use head movement (slipping and bobbing) and footwork to avoid strikes.

4. Counterattacks:

• **Timing**: Focus on timing your counterattacks immediately after defending against an opponent's strike.

Techniques:

• **Counter Punches**: Respond to incoming punches with a quick strike.

• **Counter Kicks**: When your opponent kicks, respond with a kick or strike before they can retract.

5. Takedowns and Throws:

• **Utilizing Grabs**: Secure your opponent's limbs to set up for takedowns or throws.

• **Body Control**: Use body mechanics to leverage your weight and throw your opponent to the ground or off balance.

6. Clinching:

• **Close Combat**: Engage in clinch fighting to control your opponent's movements, setting up for knee strikes or throws.

• **Technique**: Secure your opponent's head or body with your arms while maintaining a strong base to avoid being thrown.

7. Conditioning Techniques:

• **Combination Drills**: Practice various combinations of strikes and movements to improve speed and reaction times.

• **Sparring Drills**: Work with a partner on specific techniques, like counters or defensive movements, to build muscle memory and adaptability.

Sparring Strategies:

• **Stay Relaxed**: Maintain a calm and relaxed demeanor to improve focus and reaction time.

• **Control Distance**: Use footwork to control the distance between you and your opponent, maximizing your striking range while minimizing theirs.

• **Read Your Opponent**: Pay attention to your opponent's movements and patterns to anticipate their actions and create openings for your attacks.

• **Mix Up Techniques**: Vary your strikes and techniques to keep your opponent guessing and create opportunities for successful hits.

- **Know When to Engage or Retreat**: Understand when to commit to an attack and when to back off to avoid danger.

By mastering these sparring techniques and strategies in SIBPALKI, practitioners can develop their skills in a practical context, enhancing their ability to defend themselves and effectively engage in combat. Sparring serves as a critical component of martial arts training, providing valuable experience in applying techniques under pressure while fostering growth and improvement.

Strategy And Mindset In Sparring

Strategy and mindset are critical components of effective sparring in SIBPALKI. Developing a strategic approach and a focused mindset can significantly enhance a practitioner's performance and overall experience during sparring sessions.

Here's an overview of key strategies and mindset considerations for sparring:

Key Strategies in Sparring

Establish Goals:

• **Define Objectives**: Set specific goals for each sparring session, such as improving particular techniques, working on defensive skills, or testing new strategies.

• **Focus on Learning**: Approach sparring as an opportunity to learn rather than solely as a competition.

Read the Opponent:

• **Observe Patterns**: Pay attention to your opponent's movements, strikes, and tendencies to anticipate their next actions.

• **Adjust Accordingly**: Be prepared to adjust your strategy based on what you observe. For example, if your opponent favors certain strikes, develop counters to those.

Control Distance and Timing:

• **Distance Management**: Use footwork to maintain the appropriate distance for your attacks while keeping your opponent at bay.

• **Timing**: Develop an awareness of when to strike, defend, or evade based on the rhythm of the sparring session.

Incorporate Feints:

• **Deception**: Use feints to mislead your opponent into reacting to non-threatening strikes, creating openings for real attacks.

• **Set Traps**: Create scenarios where your opponent overcommits, allowing you to counter effectively.

Mix Techniques:

• **Variety**: Employ a combination of punches, kicks, and grappling techniques to keep your opponent guessing and create opportunities for successful strikes.

• **Unpredictability**: Avoid being predictable in your attacks to increase your chances of landing strikes.

Maintain Control:

• **Stay Calm**: Keep a level head and avoid becoming overly aggressive or emotional during sparring. This helps maintain clarity in decision-making.

• **Defensive Awareness**: Always be aware of your own defense, even while attacking, to avoid leaving yourself vulnerable.

Adapt and Evolve:

• **Feedback Loop**: Use each sparring session as a chance to learn. After sparring, reflect on what worked well and what could be improved.

• **Be Open to Change**: Adjust your strategies based on your experiences and the lessons learned from each sparring partner.

<u>**Mindset Considerations**</u>

Confidence:

• **Self-Belief**: Cultivate a sense of confidence in your skills and techniques, which can help reduce anxiety during sparring.

• **Positive Visualization**: Before sparring, visualize successful techniques and scenarios to enhance confidence and mental readiness.

Focus:

• **Present Moment Awareness**: Stay present and focused during sparring, avoiding distractions that can lead to mistakes.

• **Mindfulness**: Practice mindfulness techniques to enhance concentration, making it easier to read your opponent and respond appropriately.

Resilience:

• **Embrace Challenges**: Accept that sparring can be difficult and that setbacks are part of the learning process.

• **Learn from Mistakes**: View mistakes as opportunities for growth and improvement, rather than as failures.

Humility:

• **Stay Grounded**: Recognize that there is always room for improvement, no matter how skilled you become.

• **Respect Opponents**: Acknowledge the abilities of your sparring partners and learn from their strengths.

Enjoyment:

• **Have Fun**: Approach sparring with a mindset of enjoyment and exploration. This positive attitude can lead to a more productive training experience.

• **Cultivate Passion**: Foster a genuine interest in learning and improving, which can enhance motivation and engagement during sparring sessions.

By incorporating these strategies and mindset considerations, SIBPALKI practitioners can enhance their sparring experience, develop their skills, and foster a deeper understanding of martial arts. A strategic approach combined with a positive and focused mindset creates an environment conducive to learning, growth, and overall success in sparring.

CHAPTER 4: ADVANCED TECHNIQUES

Weapon Training

Weapon training is a vital aspect of SIBPALKI, enhancing practitioners' skills, coordination, and understanding of combat dynamics. The use of weapons in martial arts not only improves technique but also promotes discipline, respect, and situational awareness. Here's an overview of key components of weapon training in SIBPALKI:

Key Weapons in SIBPALKI

• **Staff (Bong)**: A long, wooden staff used for striking, blocking, and thrusting.

Techniques: Includes strikes (overhead, side, thrust), blocks, and spins. Practitioners learn to use footwork to maintain distance and control.

- **Sword (Geom)**: A traditional weapon emphasizing precision, speed, and control.

Techniques: Includes cutting, thrusting, and defensive movements. Practitioners learn to balance offense and defense while maintaining proper posture.

- **Dagger (Jangum)**: A short blade used for close-quarters combat.

Techniques: Focus on slashing, stabbing, and disarming techniques. Practitioners learn to navigate tight spaces and engage opponents effectively.

- **Nunchaku**: A pair of connected sticks that require coordination and fluidity.

Techniques: Includes strikes, spins, and locks. Training emphasizes rhythm, control, and the ability to transition between offensive and defensive movements.

• **Chain Whip (Sa Dae)**: A flexible weapon that requires skill and timing.

Techniques: Includes striking, entangling, and disarming. Practitioners learn to control the whip's movements and utilize its reach.

Training Techniques

Fundamentals:

• **Grip and Stance**: Proper grip and stance are crucial for effective weapon use. Practitioners learn to hold the weapon correctly and maintain a balanced stance.

• **Basic Movements**: Start with basic movements, including strikes, blocks, and footwork, to build a solid foundation.

Forms and Patterns (Hyung):

• **Choreographed Sequences**: Practitioners learn specific forms that incorporate various techniques, helping to develop muscle memory and fluidity.

• **Solo and Partner Drills**: Forms can be practiced solo or with a partner to enhance timing and synchronization.

Sparring with Weapons:

• **Controlled Sparring**: Engaging in controlled sparring with weapons helps practitioners apply techniques in a dynamic setting.

• **Rules and Safety**: Emphasize safety gear and rules to prevent injuries during sparring sessions.

Disarming Techniques:

• **Technique Development**: Practitioners learn techniques for disarming an opponent while maintaining control of their own weapon.

• **Situational Awareness**: Emphasize the importance of understanding distance and timing to effectively disarm an opponent.

Conditioning:

• **Strength and Flexibility**: Incorporate conditioning exercises to build strength, flexibility, and endurance, essential for effective weapon use.

• **Coordination Drills**: Focus on drills that enhance hand-eye coordination and reflexes, crucial for mastering weapon techniques.

Safety Considerations:

• **Protective Gear**: Wear appropriate protective gear, such as gloves, eye protection, and padding, when practicing with weapons to minimize injury risk.

Controlled Environment: Practice in a controlled environment, ensuring sufficient space and safety measures are in place.

Supervision: Always train under the supervision of a qualified instructor who can provide guidance and ensure safety during weapon training.

Weapon training in SIBPALKI enhances practitioners' overall martial arts skills, including coordination, timing, and situational awareness. By focusing on foundational techniques, forms, and sparring, practitioners can develop a comprehensive understanding of weapon dynamics while promoting discipline and respect within their training.

Advanced Sparring Techniques

Advanced sparring techniques in SIBPALKI are designed to enhance a practitioner's skills, timing, and strategy in dynamic sparring situations. These techniques build upon foundational skills and introduce more complex maneuvers to improve overall effectiveness in sparring. Here's an overview of key advanced sparring techniques:

Key Advanced Sparring Techniques

Combination Striking:

- **Multi-Strike Combinations**: Develop sequences that integrate various strikes (punches, kicks, knees) to overwhelm your opponent.

• **Example**: A common combination might include a jab followed by a cross, then a low kick to disrupt the opponent's balance.

Feinting and Deception:

• **Feints**: Use feints to mislead your opponent, drawing them into a reaction before executing a real attack.

• **Example**: Feint a high punch to bait a block, then deliver a low kick.

Angles and Off-Balancing:

• **Creating Angles**: Move off the centerline to create advantageous angles for strikes and avoid direct counters.

• **Off-Balancing**: Use techniques to disrupt your opponent's balance, making them vulnerable to follow-up strikes or takedowns.

Advanced Kicking Techniques:

• **Jumping and Spinning Kicks**: Incorporate jumping or spinning kicks to surprise your opponent and deliver powerful strikes.

• **Example**: A jumping roundhouse kick or a spinning back kick can create openings for strikes while adding flair to your technique.

Counterattacking:

• **Read and React**: Focus on reading your opponent's movements to set up effective counterattacks. Timing is crucial.

• **Example**: When an opponent throws a punch, slip to the side and deliver a counter punch simultaneously.

Close-Quarter Combat:

• **Clinching Techniques**: Learn to engage in close combat, utilizing knees, elbows, and grappling techniques effectively.

• **Example**: From a clinch, deliver knee strikes to the body or head while maintaining control.

Combination Defense and Attack:

• **Defensive Techniques as Offense**: Integrate defensive moves into your offensive strategy. For example, use a block to create an opening for a counter strike.

• **Example**: Block an incoming kick and immediately deliver a counter kick to the same leg.

Utilizing Distance:

• **Maintaining Range**: Develop a keen sense of distance to keep opponents at bay while being ready to engage.

• **Closing the Gap**: Use explosive footwork to close the distance quickly when an opportunity arises.

Mental Sparring:

• **Mindset Techniques**: Focus on mental preparation, visualization, and strategic thinking to enhance performance during sparring.

• **Example**: Visualize potential scenarios and your responses to them before sparring sessions to improve reaction time.

Situational Sparring:

• **Specific Scenarios**: Practice sparring in specific situations, such as defending against a wall or in a confined space, to develop adaptability.

• **Example**: Engage in drills that simulate being pressured against the ropes or in a corner.

Incorporating Advanced Techniques:

• **Partner Drills**: Work with a partner to practice advanced techniques, focusing on timing and control to minimize the risk of injury.

• **Sparring Matches**: Regularly engage in sparring matches that emphasize the use of advanced techniques, allowing you to apply them in real-time.

- **Feedback and Analysis**: After each sparring session, analyze performance with your instructor or partner to identify strengths and areas for improvement.

- **Video Analysis**: Record sparring sessions and review them to identify patterns, techniques, and areas that need work.

Mastering advanced sparring techniques in SIBPALKI allows practitioners to enhance their skills, adaptability, and overall effectiveness in combat situations. By focusing on combination striking, feinting, counterattacking, and situational awareness, practitioners can elevate their sparring game and develop a more comprehensive understanding of martial arts dynamics.

Self-Defense Applications

Self-defense applications in SIBPALKI focus on practical techniques and strategies that practitioners can use to protect themselves in real-life situations. These applications emphasize awareness, prevention, and effective responses to various threats. Here's an overview of key self-defense applications in SIBPALKI:

Key Self-Defense Principles

Awareness and Prevention:

• **Situational Awareness**: Develop the ability to assess your surroundings and identify potential threats before they escalate. This includes being aware of escape routes and potential exits.

• **De-escalation**: Utilize verbal skills and body language to defuse potential confrontations. Avoid escalating situations whenever possible.

Physical Conditioning:

• **Strength and Agility**: Maintain physical fitness to improve your ability to respond quickly in self-defense situations.

• **Endurance Training**: Build stamina to ensure you can react effectively in prolonged confrontations.

Core Self-Defense Techniques

Basic Strikes:

• **Punches and Elbows**: Use straight punches, hooks, and elbow strikes to target vulnerable areas (e.g., the nose, jaw, or solar plexus).

- **Knees and Kicks**: Deliver knee strikes to the groin or kicks to the legs to create space and disable an attacker.

Defensive Maneuvers:

- **Blocks and Parries**: Use blocking techniques to deflect incoming strikes and parry punches to create openings for counterattacks.

- **Evading**: Incorporate head movement and footwork to avoid strikes and reposition yourself for a better angle of attack.

Joint Locks and Controls:

- **Wrist Locks and Arm Bars**: Apply joint locks to immobilize or control an assailant's movement, providing an opportunity to escape.

• **Choke Holds**: Use choke holds cautiously, focusing on controlling the attacker rather than causing harm.

Takedowns and Throws:

• **Leveraging Body Weight**: Use an opponent's momentum against them to execute takedowns or throws, especially in close-quarter situations.

• **Balance Disruption**: Techniques that off-balance the attacker can help you gain control and escape.

Ground Defense:

• **Defensive Positioning**: Learn techniques to maintain control or escape if you find yourself on the ground.

• **Guard Positions**: Understand how to use guard positions to defend against an attacker while looking for escape opportunities.

Strategies for Self-Defense:

• **Target Vulnerable Areas**: Focus on striking vulnerable areas of an attacker's body, such as the eyes, throat, groin, or knees, to maximize the effectiveness of your defense.

• **Escape Over Engagement**: The primary goal of self-defense is to escape, not to engage in prolonged combat. Use techniques to create distance and get away from the situation.

• **Adapt to the Situation**: Assess the specific situation and adapt your response accordingly. Different threats may require different techniques and strategies.

- **Practice with Realism**: Engage in scenario-based training to practice self-defense techniques in a controlled environment that mimics real-life situations.

- **Use of Environment**: Be aware of your surroundings and utilize objects around you as potential tools for defense (e.g., using a bag to block an attack or throwing objects to create a distraction).

<u>Mental Preparedness:</u>

- **Confidence**: Build confidence in your ability to defend yourself through regular practice and training. A confident mindset can deter potential attackers.

- **Decision Making**: Practice making quick decisions in high-pressure situations. This includes knowing when to engage and when to escape.

• **Calmness Under Pressure**: Train to remain calm during confrontations. A clear mind can help you think strategically and react effectively.

Self-defense applications in SIBPALKI empower practitioners with the skills, techniques, and mindset necessary to protect themselves in various situations. By focusing on awareness, practical techniques, and mental preparedness, practitioners can enhance their ability to respond effectively to threats while prioritizing safety and escape. Regular training in self-defense not only builds physical skills but also instills confidence and resilience in everyday life.

CHAPTER 5: TRAINING AND CONDITIONING

Physical Conditioning For SIBPALKI

Physical conditioning is crucial for practitioners of SIBPALKI to enhance their overall performance, strength, agility, and endurance. A well-rounded conditioning program supports the execution of techniques, improves recovery, and reduces the risk of injury. Here's a comprehensive guide to physical conditioning for SIBPALKI:

Components of Physical Conditioning

Cardiovascular Endurance:

• **Importance**: Increases stamina and the ability to sustain high-intensity activity during training and sparring.

Exercises:

• **Running**: Long-distance and interval running improve cardiovascular health and endurance.

• **Jump Rope**: Enhances footwork, coordination, and cardiovascular endurance.

• **Cycling**: Low-impact option for building endurance and leg strength.

Strength Training:

• **Importance**: Builds muscle strength and power, essential for striking, blocking, and grappling.

Exercises:

• **Weightlifting**: Focus on compound movements such as squats, deadlifts, and bench presses to build overall strength.

- **Bodyweight Exercises**: Push-ups, pull-ups, and dips enhance upper body strength without the need for equipment.

- **Resistance Bands**: Useful for strengthening smaller muscles and improving flexibility.

Flexibility and Mobility:

- **Importance**: Reduces the risk of injury and enhances the range of motion necessary for executing techniques.

Exercises:

- **Dynamic Stretching**: Perform before workouts to warm up muscles and improve mobility (e.g., leg swings, arm circles).

- **Static Stretching**: Perform after workouts to increase flexibility (e.g., hamstring stretches, hip flexor stretches).

- **Yoga**: Incorporates flexibility, balance, and core strength, beneficial for overall body conditioning.

Agility and Coordination:

- **Importance**: Enhances the ability to move quickly and efficiently, crucial for effective footwork and technique execution.

Exercises:

- **Ladder Drills**: Improve foot speed and coordination.

- **Cone Drills**: Enhance agility and the ability to change directions quickly.

- **Plyometrics**: Jumping exercises (box jumps, burpees) develop explosive power and coordination.

Core Strength:

• **Importance**: Supports balance, stability, and power generation in martial arts movements.

Exercises:

•   **Planks**: Strengthen the entire core, including the abdominals and lower back.

•   **Russian Twists**: Improve rotational strength, important for twisting motions in strikes and throws.

• **Leg Raises**: Target the lower abs and hip flexors.

Sample Conditioning Routine

Warm-Up (10-15 minutes):

• **Dynamic Stretching**: Leg swings, arm circles, hip rotations.

• **Jump Rope**: 3 minutes to increase heart rate and warm up muscles.

Cardiovascular Training (20-30 minutes):

• **Interval Running**: Alternate between 1 minute of sprinting and 2 minutes of jogging.

• **Cycling**: Steady-state cycling at a moderate pace.

Strength Training (30-45 minutes):

• **Compound Lifts**: Squats, deadlifts, bench presses (3 sets of 8-12 reps).

• **Bodyweight Exercises**: Push-ups, pull-ups, dips (3 sets of max reps).

Agility and Plyometrics (15-20 minutes):

• **Ladder Drills**: 3-4 different patterns, 2 sets each.

- **Cone Drills**: Shuttle runs, side-to-side hops.

- **Plyometrics**: Box jumps, burpees (3 sets of 10 reps).

Core Training (10-15 minutes):

- **Planks**: 3 sets of 1 minute each.

- **Russian Twists**: 3 sets of 20 twists.

- **Leg Raises**: 3 sets of 15 reps.

Cool Down (10-15 minutes):

- **Static Stretching**: Hold each stretch for 30 seconds to 1 minute.

- **Deep Breathing**: Practice deep breathing to relax muscles and promote recovery.

Recovery and Injury Prevention

• **Proper Nutrition**: Fuel your body with a balanced diet rich in proteins, carbohydrates, and healthy fats to support muscle growth and recovery.

• **Hydration**: Maintain adequate hydration before, during, and after training sessions.

• **Rest**: Ensure sufficient rest between intense training sessions to allow muscles to recover and prevent overtraining.

• **Injury Prevention**: Listen to your body and address any pain or discomfort immediately to prevent injuries. Incorporate regular mobility work and foam rolling to keep muscles supple.

Effective physical conditioning for SIBPALKI involves a comprehensive approach that includes cardiovascular endurance, strength training, flexibility, agility, and core strength. By following a well-rounded conditioning routine, practitioners can enhance their performance, reduce the risk of injury, and improve their overall martial arts capabilities. Regular training, combined with proper recovery and injury prevention strategies, will support long-term success and well-being in martial arts practice.

Mental conditioning and focus are critical aspects of SIBPALKI, as they enhance a practitioner's ability to stay calm, make strategic decisions, and maintain peak performance during training and combat. Here's an in-depth guide to mental conditioning and focus techniques for SIBPALKI practitioners:

<u>Key Components of Mental Conditioning</u>

Mindfulness and Meditation:

• **Importance**: Develops a calm, focused mind, reducing stress and improving concentration.

Techniques:

• **Breathing Exercises**: Practice deep, diaphragmatic breathing to calm the mind and body. For example, inhale for four counts, hold for four counts, and exhale for four counts.

• **Meditation**: Spend 10-15 minutes daily in seated meditation, focusing on your breath or a mantra to cultivate inner stillness.

Visualization:

• **Importance**: Enhances mental rehearsal of techniques, builds confidence, and prepares the mind for performance.

Techniques:

• **Positive Visualization**: Visualize yourself successfully executing techniques, overcoming challenges, and achieving your goals.

• **Scenario Visualization**: Imagine different sparring or self-defense scenarios and mentally practice your responses.

Goal Setting:

• **Importance**: Provides direction, motivation, and a sense of achievement.

Techniques:

• **SMART Goals**: Set Specific, Measurable, Achievable, Relevant, and Time-bound goals. Break long-term goals into smaller, manageable milestones.

• **Regular Review**: Periodically review and adjust your goals to reflect progress and new aspirations.

Positive Self-Talk:

• **Importance**: Builds confidence and resilience, countering negative thoughts that can hinder performance.

Techniques:

• **Affirmations**: Use positive affirmations to reinforce self-belief. For example, "I am strong and capable" or "I can handle any challenge."

• **Reframing**: Reframe negative thoughts into positive or constructive ones. For example, change "I can't do this" to "I will find a way to do this."

Stress Management:

• **Importance**: Helps maintain composure and effectiveness under pressure.

Techniques:

• **Progressive Muscle Relaxation**: Tense and relax different muscle groups to release physical and mental tension.

- **Time Management**: Organize your schedule to balance training, rest, and personal life, reducing overall stress.

Enhancing Focus

Concentration Drills:

- **Importance**: Improves the ability to maintain attention during training and combat.

Techniques:

- **Focused Training**: Practice techniques with full attention, avoiding distractions. Use a timer to train in focused intervals (e.g., 25 minutes of focused practice followed by a 5-minute break).

- **Mental Drills**: Engage in activities that require sustained focus, such as reading, puzzles, or memory games.

Routine Development:

• **Importance**: Establishes consistency and prepares the mind for training.

Techniques:

• **Pre-Training Rituals**: Develop a routine before training sessions, such as specific warm-up exercises or mental preparation techniques.

• **Consistency**: Train at the same time and place whenever possible to create a stable environment for focused practice.

Flow State:

• **Importance**: Achieves peak performance by being fully immersed in the activity.

Techniques:

• **Challenge-Skill Balance**: Engage in tasks that are challenging yet match your skill level to maintain engagement and avoid boredom or frustration.

• **Clear Goals and Feedback**: Set clear, immediate goals and seek feedback to stay focused and motivated.

Application in Training and Sparring

Focused Sparring:

Techniques:

• **Set Intentions**: Before sparring, set specific intentions or goals for the session, such as improving a particular technique or strategy.

• **Reflective Practice**: After sparring, reflect on what went well and what can be improved. Use this reflection to focus future training sessions.

Mental Warm-Up:

Techniques:

• **Visualization**: Spend a few minutes before training visualizing your techniques and goals for the session.

• **Breathing Exercises**: Use breathing techniques to calm the mind and prepare for focused training.

Adapting to Pressure:

Techniques:

• **Simulated Pressure**: Practice under simulated pressure conditions to build resilience. For example, spar with a more experienced partner or in front of an audience.

- **Mindfulness in Action**: Practice staying present and focused during high-stress training scenarios to improve your ability to handle real-life pressure.

Mental conditioning and focus are essential for SIBPALKI practitioners to excel in training, sparring, and real-life self-defense situations. By incorporating mindfulness, visualization, goal setting, positive self-talk, and stress management techniques, practitioners can enhance their mental resilience and concentration. Regular practice of these techniques will lead to improved performance, greater confidence, and a deeper understanding of the mental aspects of martial arts.

Injury Prevention And Recovery

Injury prevention and recovery are vital components of SIBPALKI training, ensuring that practitioners can train safely and effectively while minimizing downtime due to injuries. Here's an in-depth guide to strategies for injury prevention and effective recovery practices:

Injury Prevention Strategies

Proper Warm-Up and Cool-Down:

• **Warm-Up**: Always start with a thorough warm-up to increase blood flow, loosen muscles, and prepare the body for intense activity.

• **Dynamic Stretching**: Incorporate dynamic movements like leg swings, arm circles, and hip rotations.

• **Light Cardio**: Engage in light jogging or jump rope for 5-10 minutes.

• **Cool-Down**: After training, cool down with static stretching to relax muscles and improve flexibility.

• **Static Stretching**: Hold each stretch for 20-30 seconds, focusing on major muscle groups.

Proper Technique:

• **Training**: Always focus on proper form and technique to avoid unnecessary strain and injury.

• **Supervision**: Train under the guidance of a qualified instructor to ensure techniques are performed correctly.

Gradual Progression:

•   **Incremental Increases**: Gradually increase the intensity, duration, and complexity of your training to allow the body to adapt.

• **Listen to Your Body**: Pay attention to signs of fatigue or discomfort and avoid pushing through pain.

Strength and Conditioning:

• **Balanced Training**: Incorporate strength training to support muscles and joints. Focus on overall body strength, not just martial arts-specific muscles.

• **Core Strength**: A strong core provides stability and reduces the risk of injuries.

Protective Gear:

• **Use Appropriate Gear**: Wear protective equipment such as mouthguards, gloves, shin guards, and headgear during sparring and intense training sessions.

• **Check Equipment**: Regularly inspect gear for wear and tear and replace it as necessary.

Hydration and Nutrition:

• **Stay Hydrated**: Drink plenty of water before, during, and after training to maintain hydration levels.

• **Balanced Diet**: Consume a diet rich in proteins, carbohydrates, healthy fats, vitamins, and minerals to support muscle recovery and overall health.

Rest and Recovery:

• **Adequate Sleep**: Ensure you get sufficient sleep to allow your body to recover and repair.

• **Rest Days**: Incorporate rest days into your training schedule to prevent overtraining and allow for recovery.

<u>**Recovery Techniques**</u>

Immediate Post-Injury Care:

• **R.I.C.E Method**: For acute injuries, follow the Rest, Ice, Compression, and Elevation protocol.

• **Rest**: Avoid using the injured area.

• **Ice**: Apply ice to reduce swelling and pain.

• **Compression**: Use an elastic bandage to provide support and reduce swelling.

• **Elevation**: Elevate the injured limb above heart level to reduce swelling.

Physical Therapy and Rehabilitation:

• **Consult a Professional**: Seek the guidance of a physiotherapist or sports medicine specialist for injury-specific rehabilitation exercises.

• **Follow a Rehab Plan**: Adhere to a structured rehabilitation plan to ensure proper healing and prevent re-injury.

Active Recovery:

• **Light Activity**: Engage in low-impact activities like walking, swimming, or yoga to maintain mobility and circulation without over-stressing the injured area.

- **Gentle Stretching**: Perform gentle stretching exercises to maintain flexibility and prevent stiffness.

Massage and Foam Rolling:

- **Massage Therapy**: Regular massages can help relieve muscle tension, improve circulation, and promote relaxation.

- **Foam Rolling**: Use a foam roller to release muscle tightness and improve blood flow to the muscles.

Heat Therapy:

- **Heat Packs**: Apply heat packs to sore or stiff muscles to promote relaxation and improve blood flow.

- **Warm Baths**: Taking warm baths, possibly with Epsom salts, can help soothe muscles and reduce soreness.

Hydration and Nutrition:

• **Post-Training Nutrition**: Consume protein-rich foods or shakes after training to aid in muscle repair and recovery.

• **Anti-Inflammatory Foods**: Include foods rich in omega-3 fatty acids, antioxidants, and vitamins to reduce inflammation and support recovery.

Monitoring and Professional Care

Regular Check-Ups:

• **Medical Evaluations**: Periodically visit a healthcare professional for assessments to catch potential issues early.

• **Specialist Consultation**: Consult specialists such as sports medicine doctors, chiropractors, or physiotherapists when necessary.

Monitoring Progress:

• **Keep a Training Log**: Document your training routines, any pain or discomfort, and recovery progress.

• **Adjust as Needed**: Modify training intensity and techniques based on feedback from your body and professionals.

Injury prevention and recovery are essential for sustaining long-term martial arts practice. By incorporating proper warm-ups, strength training, and protective gear, you can minimize the risk of injuries. In the event of an injury, following immediate care protocols, engaging in active recovery, and seeking professional guidance will aid in effective recovery. Balancing training intensity with adequate rest, nutrition, and hydration further supports overall health and performance in SIBPALKI.

Conclusion

In SIBPALKI, achieving and maintaining peak physical and mental condition is essential for effective training, performance, and long-term practice. A holistic approach that includes proper physical conditioning, mental focus, injury prevention, and effective recovery strategies ensures that practitioners can train safely and consistently while minimizing downtime due to injuries.

Key Takeaways:

• **Physical Conditioning**: Emphasize a balanced regimen of cardiovascular endurance, strength training, flexibility, agility, and core strength to enhance overall performance and reduce injury risk.

• **Mental Conditioning and Focus**: Cultivate mindfulness, visualization, goal setting, positive self-talk, and stress management techniques to improve concentration, resilience, and decision-making during training and sparring.

• **Injury Prevention**: Prioritize proper warm-up and cool-down routines, use correct techniques, gradually progress training intensity, incorporate strength and conditioning exercises, wear protective gear, and maintain hydration and nutrition.

• **Recovery Strategies**: Implement immediate post-injury care using the R.I.C.E method, follow structured rehabilitation plans, engage in active recovery through light activities and stretching, utilize massage and foam rolling, and apply heat therapy to soothe muscles.

• **Professional Care and Monitoring**: Regular check-ups with healthcare professionals and specialists, along with careful monitoring of training routines and recovery progress, ensure that potential issues are addressed promptly and effectively.

By integrating these components, SIBPALKI practitioners can maximize their training outcomes, maintain their health and well-being, and continue to grow and excel in their martial arts journey. The commitment to both physical and mental conditioning, along with a proactive approach to injury prevention and recovery, lays a strong foundation for sustained success and enjoyment in SIBPALKI.

Glossary of Terms:

- **SIBPALKI**: A traditional Korean martial art focusing on techniques and principles for practical combat and self-defense.

- **Martial Arts**: Various forms of combat practices that are performed for a variety of reasons including self-defense, military and law enforcement applications, competition, physical fitness, mental and spiritual development.

- **Hwa**: Harmony; the principle of blending and adapting to an opponent's movements.

- **Won**: Circularity; the use of circular movements to deflect attacks and create openings.

- **Yu**: Flow; the concept of fluidity in movement and technique execution.

- **Ki**: Internal energy; the vital life force that is cultivated and used in martial arts practices.

- **Juchum Seogi**: Horse stance; a wide, low stance used for stability and power.

- **Ap Seogi**: Front stance; a stance with one leg forward and the other back, used for forward movement and attacks.

- **Dwi Seogi**: Back stance; a stance with most weight on the back leg, used for defense and evasion.

- **Ap Chagi**: Front kick; a basic kicking technique aimed at the opponent's torso or head.

- **Dwi Chagi**: Back kick; a powerful kick delivered by turning the body and striking with the heel.

- **Sidang Chagi**: Side kick; a kick delivered to the opponent's side with the heel or blade of the foot.

- **Dan Jun Ho Hup**: Abdominal breathing; a method of breathing deeply into the abdomen to generate power and control.

- **Hap Gi**: Breathing coordination; synchronizing breath with movement to enhance technique and energy flow.

- **Jireugi**: Punching; delivering strikes with a closed fist.

- **Chigi**: Striking; various hand strikes, including open-hand techniques.

- **Makgi**: Blocking; using the arms to deflect or stop an opponent's attack.

- Kicking Techniques

- **Yeop Chagi**: Side kick; delivering a powerful kick to the side of the opponent.

- **Dollyo Chagi**: Roundhouse kick; a circular kick aimed at the opponent's head or torso.

- **Neryo Chagi**: Axe kick; a downward strike with the heel.

- **Bakkat Makgi**: Outer block; a technique used to deflect an opponent's attack to the outside.

- **Japgi**: Grappling; techniques used to grab and control an opponent.

- **Ttakgi**: Throwing; techniques used to unbalance and throw an opponent to the ground.

- **Kwan Jul**: Joint lock; techniques used to control or incapacitate an opponent by locking their joints.

- **Danggi**: Holding; securing an opponent in a fixed position.

- **Paljul**: Arm lock; a technique that targets the opponent's elbow or shoulder joints.

- **Kyogi**: Sparring; practicing combat techniques against a live opponent in a controlled setting.

- **Matsogi**: Matched sparring; structured sparring with pre-arranged techniques and movements.

- **Mok Geom**: Wooden sword; used for practicing sword techniques.

- **Jang Bong**: Long staff; a traditional Korean weapon used for striking and blocking.

- **Dan Bong**: Short staff; used for close-range combat and striking techniques.

- **Hyeong**: Forms; pre-arranged sequences of movements that simulate combat scenarios.

- **Gongkyok**: Offensive techniques; various attacks designed to defeat an opponent.

- **Banguh**: Defensive techniques; methods used to protect oneself from attacks.

- **Musa**: Warrior spirit; the mental attitude of courage, determination, and resilience.

- **Seon**: Zen; a state of meditative focus and mindfulness in practice and combat.

- **Jungeui**: Flexibility; the ability to move joints through their full range of motion.

- **Cheolhap**: Coordination; the harmonious integration of different body movements.

- **Gangseong**: Strength; the ability to exert force for performing techniques effectively.

Learning these definitions will help you study and practice SIBPALKI, a traditional martial art, to a deeper level.

ABOUT THE AUTHOR:

Kameron Jalen, an author, frequently employs his profound comprehension of human nature and personal experiences to investigate a diverse array of themes in his writing. His compositions may encompass instructional materials, non-fiction, or fiction, which demonstrate his capacity to articulate intricate concepts in a manner that is both engaging and comprehensible. Jalen's objective in his writing is to motivate and inspire readers by imparting knowledge on the significance of personal development, self-discipline, and resilience.

Kameron Jalen is also a dedicated martial arts practitioner, having trained in a variety of disciplines. His proficiency in martial arts is not only indicative of his physical abilities, but also underscores the philosophical and cerebral components of the discipline. He is likely to promote the advantages of martial arts in the development of focus, discipline, and confidence, and he may conduct seminars or teach classes to disseminate his expertise. He integrates the principles of hard work and perseverance into both his writing and teaching, as evidenced by his martial arts journey.

Kameron Jalen has a Ph.D. in a pertinent discipline from a prestigious university in the United States, in addition to his creative and physical activities. His academic education equips him with a robust foundation for his writing and teaching, enabling him to approach subjects with a critical and analytical perspective. His scholarly work and research may concentrate on the social implications of martial arts, human behavior, or psychology, thereby contributing to both academic discourse and practical applications.

Kameron Jalen possesses an uncommon combination of academic rigor, physical prowess, and creativity. He remains a source of inspiration and influence for those in his vicinity, motivating them to pursue their interests and aspire for excellence in all aspects of life because of his diverse talents. Jalen is dedicated to the promotion of personal and professional development, whether through his academic lectures, martial arts classes, or publications.

THE END